Trauma
Healing
Action
Steps
For
Veterans

*

Forgiveness

Reverend Mike Wanner

Table of Contents

Dedication

This book is dedicated to all those who have served to defend the United States of America and their families who have served also by missing them during their service and some forever. These valiant citizens have given freely in the pursuit of the noble goals specified in the Declaration of Independence and the Constitution of The United States and all the amendments thereto.

Special recognition is offered to those who have been killed in the service of our country. The citizens now and future citizens of the United States of America will be forever in their debt. May all who have served and their families be blessed in the now and the forever AND SO IT IS!

Special recognition is offered to those who have been injured in the service of our country. The citizens now and future citizens of the United States of America will be forever in their debt. The injured warriors of our nation have performed well a duty and this writing is offered to help mitigate some of the emotional turmoil that may still reside within those valiant ones. May each of them and their families be blessed in all ways in the now and the forever AND SO IT IS!

It is the intent of this work to help Veterans to reclaim their power after their military service is complete.

May All who Read this book be Blessed AND SO IT IS!

Reverend Mike Wanner

Acknowledgements

I would like to acknowledge the support of the following beings:

Ceil Nuyianes is an Earth Angel who started as a student of mine in Reiki and developed into a friend whose book industry expertise helped guide me in many ways.

Mary E. Jay who has been an inspiration.

Nancy Russell was my Integrated Energy Therapy Master Instructor who introduced me to Angel Ariel and the methodology of Heartlinking with the Angels to facilitate the clearing of stuffed emotions and cellular memory.

Stevan Thayer was my Integrated Energy Therapy Master Instructor Trainer who taught me how to teach others How to Heal with The Energy of Angels.

My Reiki Masters were Rita Hildenbrandt, Hannelore Goodwin, Gary Jirauch, Tom Rigler, Patrick Zigler, Hiroshi Doi, Chiyoko Yamaguchi, Tadao Yamaguchi and especially the founder of Komyo Kai Reiki Reverend Hyakuten Inamoto Otto.

Reverend Ethel Lomardi who taught me the healing power of viewing people as pure light.

Archangels Michael - the Protector, Gabriel - the Communicator,
Raphael- the Healer and the legions of Angels that help the healing process for all.

Chapter 1

The Toxicity of Guilt

The energy of guilt whether it is from a deliberate or required action can be detrimental to the peace and harmony of the one holding it. It may seem as if there will never again be a circumstance where one can be worthy of good.

Guilt is like hazardous waste as it can hurt everyone it comes in contact with and spread like a contagious disease to innocent victims that simply are in the way of the flow. Everyone associated with someone who carries the guilt burden can be hurt.

Guilt is like garbage from the life that you have lived through. While there is no need to keep garbage in your kitchen, there is also no need to keep guilt in your life or hold others in guilt for which they have offered amends.

Yes, "I'm sorry" only goes so far. The sentiment and delivery of the conciliatory effort can allow you to sense the depth of the feeling that brings it.

We all know the difference between sincerity and required apologies. The challenge for the receiver of any apology is to remain objective and not prejudge someone based on the past.

People can change and allowing toxic quilt to exit one's life is a tremendous step on a healing path. Forgiveness is like defusing a bomb, it can prevent a lot of future damage. The forgiver and the forgivee benefit as do all they know and interact with.

Chapter 2

Forgive Others

Many of the injustices in life that bother us the most are when something about what was done by another reminds us of any personal quilt that we may have for the same or a similar thing. While it is not easy to take responsibility for our actions, it is easy to judge others for their actions so many people are quick to blame and judge others without objectivity.

When you want to develop yourself physically, you go to a gym and do exercise with the hope that you will develop one muscle and then another and then more. You build up to the goals that you have set for yourself.

Forgiveness is like joining a gym. You have to build up to it. Being responsible for our personal healing does not come easy to any of us.

Blaming others for our failures is a sad way to try and save face. We and everyone else know who exactly is responsible for our situation.

We can build character, like building muscle, by doing what needs to be done to get through the emotional façade and own the situation that we choose. When we forgive others for any part that they had in our failure, we allow ourselves to be front and center for our own failure or success.

Forgiving others is therefore, an early step in the process of forgiving ourselves.

Chapter 3

Forgive Yourself

Veterans can be bothered by actually feeling guilty for doing what they were ordered to do and then guilty for doing what they may not have agreed needed to be done. The right or wrong may be argued but the guilt can be deep.

Deep guilt can anchor within and be problematic to heal. Even slight guilt can be disruptive to an innocent person's life.

Persons that are innocent from deliberate willful actions may feel tainted by what they were ordered to do. Finding justification may not be easy. When we can forgive ourselves for misdeeds, we can find a positive foundation upon which we can build our future life.

Forgiving oneself allows for objectivity that can really help to re-introduce a new level of possibilities that never existed before. Releasing judgment is like untying a knot in a supply line that allows the flow to go from full stop to full flow.

If others are involved, sometimes when we let go of a situation there will follow some sort of shift from the other person that will allow them to step up to the plate and be conciliatory.

Candidness

Freedom from self-blame allows a freedom where one can reassess the situation they are in. If you have forgiven all, you are beginning to get the feeling that I am talking about. If you have not forgiven all then you do not yet realize all the power that is at your disposal.

Forgiveness allows you to be free of the past so that you can enjoy the present. As long as you are trying to get even with somebody, you are not truly free to find and enjoy the blessings that God is forever showering down upon you.

Stumbling Blocks

If you reach a point where you find stumbling blocks, know that is OK. Change does not always happen overnight and you can take the time you need to get to where you want to be.

Make some notes of your immediate goals, any feelings of struggle and any perceived obstacles. Be sure to record the date and time of your notation so that you have a reference.

This would also be a good time to plan a small action step that can help take you in the direction of a goal.

Chapter 4

Are you a Victim?

When you hear yourself telling your story to others, listen to hear if the story paints you as a victim. Are you telling a story of unfairness where you are the innocent party who is victimized by others or a situation?

The retelling of the story over and over again will keep you stuck in the story that was then and it will not allow you to be in the fullness of life in the present time. Would you like to break the cycle of the past and allow yourself to fully enjoy the present and the future?

If you answered yes, then it is time for you to get busy and create the reality that you would like.

Allowing the past to simply be history is a giant step forward in the creation of your optimal future. Take some time to journal your experience.

Divide your story in to segments that can be assigned to categories. You need to know:

- The Issues
- The participants
- How things happened?
- Who did what?
- Whether options were considered?
- Repercussions

Chapter 5

Healing the Past

As you continue to move forward, be careful about your thinking and how you describe the situation to yourself and all others. For if you have accepted any culpability that you had in the situation and forgiven yourself and others then there is no need to continue to blame others and distract yourself from any guilt that might be pointed at you.

You may find it helpful to own all the experience that you had, continue to accept any responsibility that you might have had and then see yourself on the mend so that you can allow the pain to go. As you continue to reprocess and release the pain of the past, there will be a reinvigoration that eases in to your awareness. Allow yourself to observe the freshness that is coming in to your life while analyzing your worthiness to receive.

As you continue to work at polishing the diamond that you are, there will be issues that surface and cause you to rethink what you are doing. Do not let these distractions impede you. You are the creator of your own life and you are the one in the driver's seat now.

As a child, you followed the instructions of your parents. As a serviceperson, you followed the orders of your leaders.

As a veteran, you get to rethink and realign your life according to your values and beliefs. You also get to release that which was required of you and forgive yourself for following instructions that were not aligned with the peace that resides within your heart. Now is the time for you to take responsibility to be a good person.

Chapter 6

Speak about the Present

Matter of fact statements will allow you to be aware of the past but moving in to the present as you plan for the future at the same time. Acknowledge your struggles and be better than hiding from them. Power comes from the truth of the reality that you can process and accept.

Know that it is not unusual for old stuff to seep in to your statements and while it should not be a major concern, it is the type of stuff that you want to acknowledge as old, tired, history that is not currently an issue in your life. It is a good idea to write them down if you are busy so that you can revisit them later and be sure to heal them when convenient.

Do not be alarmed if there seems to be a lot of stuff at one time that comes. Treat it all the same as history which you have grown from and released into the past as you are busy in the present creating your life the way you like it.

Note-taking is a process that can be particularly helpful to grab awareness of things to revisit when you want to so that you can continue to lead your life on your timetable. Remember to come back and put out the clutter that might have built up over time. Sweep it up when you are ready and release it all.

Chapter 7

Ho‘oponopono

This is a great tool to use when doing self-polishing work. I include the Wikipedia Explanation:

"Ho‘oponopono (ho-o-pono-pono) is an <u>ancient Hawaiian</u> practice of <u>reconciliation</u> and <u>forgiveness</u>. Similar forgiveness practices were performed on islands throughout the <u>South Pacific</u>, including <u>Samoa</u>, <u>Tahiti</u> and <u>New Zealand</u>. Traditionally *ho‘oponopono* is practiced by healing priests or *kahuna lapa‘au* among family members of a person who is physically ill. Modern versions are performed within the family by a family elder, or by the individual alone."

The Four step clearing process of Ho’oponopono is very simple yet powerful when applied to all that troubles you. The practice is well represented on the internet and music is there also that can help with the practice. Please visit the various sites to learn enough to practice it with the best technique.

The concept is to avoid blaming others and ask what is it about me that is causing _____? With that said, you seek further knowing by declaring:

- I love you
- I’m Sorry
- Please forgive me
- Thank you

Anyone can practice Ho’oponopono.

I Love you

This practice goes well with forgiveness because the focus shifts to making things right and allowing oneself to realign with the universe.

The declaration of love opens oneself to all that is good and right in the universe. It can be directed broadly or specifically as you are seeing things in the moment.

Even when one is drawn to be very specific with their declaration of "I Love You", please know that there is great value in inclusiveness. The more that you can align with love for all that you perceive, the more you can acknowledge, activate, trigger, connect with and be in harmony with all that can serve the good of all within your experience and their experience.

If you think of love like rain showering subtly on a parched earth, you can begin to feel the healing value of starting to plant seeds of love in all matters that have not been optimal so that tomorrow begins a new day to grow for everything and everyone upon the earth.

Many have a tendency to think of ourselves as small and insignificant but the truth of that is the only part of us that is insignificant is that very thought. We are created in the image and likeness of God and we are instilled with great power which can bless many.

I Am Sorry

Ho'oponopono is about correcting all that we see so that it is made right. The beauty of the process that I see is in the clarity and objectivity as they merge in to a process which blends sorrow and acceptance into a coincidental reality check which allows truth to be acknowledged as part of the healing as it releases guilt.

Making things right with God and the ancestors and all concerned with a situation is a dramatic step in the direction of revitalization for all that were in any way connected to or impacted.

Please Forgive Me

Asking for forgiveness expresses the depth of our concern and regret for all that has occurred. On one hand it declares one's remorse but it is also an invitation for those affected to know the truth of our feeling after reflection on all that occurred.

The request for forgiveness acknowledges responsibility so that settlement can occur.

Thank You

Gratitude is both a show of appreciation and an indication of closure for all that has been shared.

Chapter 8

Stop Seeing the Present Thru The Past

Resist the temptation to see the present thru the filter of the pain of the past. It does not serve you. Continue to pursue a new present and future that is aligned with your wanting.

While this is easily said, doing it can be quite a bit more of a challenge as we have the habits that are familiar to us. Our autopilot starts easily to move in a certain direction according to all that is familiar to us.

To accomplish new goals, we will need new priorities, goals, tools, techniques, perceptions and the flexibility to adapt and overcome obstacles. When something is not working for us, we need the adaptability to shift in the middle of any project and channel corrective action.

Accept at the beginning that the required flexibility will be contrary to your inclinations, so it is important that you be creative and cautious about the direction that you take. Don't be afraid to stop and regroup whenever you feel that you are off course.

New options will become available as you continue to self-correct your inclinations and choose options that may be unfamiliar. New experiences can lead to finding a new level of potential for all that you wish to attract into your life.

Patience with yourself will be key to your success so resist all autopilot judging inclinations that will likely kick-in to rattle yourself and trigger self-doubt.

Chapter 9

Where Is Forgiveness Needed?

Let's take a little measurement and see what new awareness has been stimulated by the perspective that I have shared.

Who needs Forgiveness & how much is their share of responsibility that they need forgiveness for? Include all who should be on the list even if you feel that you will never be able to forgive them. This last can include many who may not be in direct contact with you and may be authority figures in some circles who have taken steps that indirectly cause a lack of ease in your circumstance.

_____

_____

_____

_____

Why do the above people need forgiveness? Be aware that there may have been a perspective shift from your original position. You are free to edit or trim the list as you go.

_____

_____

_____

_____

Be open to any rethinking about your relationships with the list as you may remember them now less harshly than your original assessment. You can accept obvious reassessments at any time.

Chapter 10

Authority Figures

There may be great conflict when it comes to authority figures in your life and their needing to be forgiven by you. While this may be more or a challenge than other areas of your life, it can still be accomplished when you arrive at a point where you can make the shift.

Do not be concerned with the level of intensity that may be required to complete a task. Know that forgiveness has a lot to offer you and some situations may require more effort.

Freedom that comes from forgiveness is worth the effort and should be pursued by all feasible measures. You will be amazed at the success that you can have by merely revisiting situations in your mind's eye and using evaluation skills that your older self may have that were not yours at the time that they occurred.

Age brings subtle increases in perspective that can be very helpful and maturity allows you to look at the whole situation without being petty and rigid. Sometimes a good laugh can be had that changes what you remember and allows a fresh assessment of the importance thereof.

The highest authority figure is of course God and s/he is often overlooked as one to forgive because the forgiveness power is in our decision to forgive and not in the expression of it. When we decide to forgive, we open like the bloom of a flower to all that is there for us. While God does not benefit directly from us uttering forgiveness, we do benefit from the decision and each effort to express it.

Chapter 11

The Innocent Ones Nearby

When guilt has been shared with any group of people, the remedy to the situation is much more difficult than the action. Young people especially can be deeply scared by violent outbursts and attacks.

Whether you or someone you know has caused an outburst of attack rage, it can take many people and a lot of time to repair the damage done. I share this not to judge or condemn but as a reality check that one can use to receive motivation to do what is needed to undo anything like that they are aware of and more importantly to discourage reoccurrences.

Forgiveness sets a new stage of expectation for a future that can be different from the past. While the sting of the memory will remain, the strength of the healing will influence not only the quality but the frequency of future good.

Positivity can also be reinforced to make clear to all that vulnerable situations are eliminated. Herein lays a struggle that can be expected in that the memory of the past could be a subtle reminder that keeps us from fully embracing all that could be in the present but awareness can also be helpful so we choose our actions wisely.

Conscious effort will be needed to diligently claim the highest joy in every minute so that goodness and peace of mind are forever present. While one can carry an umbrella for use on rainy days, it serves not to carry the umbrella in a fully open position because that can create other issues. Awareness and diligence will serve well so that the peace of each moment can be enjoyed fully.

Chapter 12

Finding Joy

Our diligence in all matters allows us to find relaxed living and peaceful relationships. As we walk within the community and share both the giving and receiving of respect and love, we allow the quality of life to continue to improve for all and in that way there can occur an amplification of the goodness for all.

Giving and receiving can be the same so there can be little effort needed to share wonderful experiences with others. Also, when sadness eventually comes there will be a sharing of the pain so that the sting is somewhat diminished.

As the saying goes, when we share our Love, we double it. When we share our pain, we cut it in half.

As a veteran, your experiences are many and you may have had more than your fair share of negativity. Please consider that it may be time for the pendulum to swing in the opposite direction and you can receive positive benefits regardless of all that has gone before.

There is an important element for you to be aware of and that is the simple fact that you must be willing to receive. This may sound like a stupid suggestion but I submit that humans are creatures of habit and many times we expect things to be a certain way and act with that expectancy in mind and then what we expect seems to happen.

Please know that active participation in the change of your expectations is a key element to you receiving your just share of everything. Adjusting your expectancy is the beginning of all that needs to change.

As you have forgiven and expect to receive a new flow of blessings, you will radiate a vibration that will output a harmonic alignment with the good that you expect and people and things aligned with that vibration will begin to show up in your life. Surprised you may be by the intensity of the change.

This change will not be all about receiving because the ebb and flow of life involves your participation. Knowing what is needed does not require effort as it can be as natural as the seasons.

Chapter 13

The Power within Your Thoughts

The intensity within your thinking has a lot of influence on the ability of your thoughts to bring you the best and the worst of everything. As you converse with others, be aware of all that comes from the depth of your emotions and also all that comes from others that is shared with you. Forgive everybody for everything.

Thoughts have a way of getting wedged in places within oneself and they can then have influence long past the time they were expressed. Awareness of these thoughts can help you to select and focus upon the ones that serve you and also help you select and release the ones whose service is no longer relevant.

Our minds are like computers that we self-program with priorities that are accurate at the time of the placement. As situations change, the appropriateness of certain programs may diminish and their benefit may pale when compared to the resources that they consume. Forgive everybody for everything.

If we are not aware of our need to reset the priorities within our minds, we can waste a lot of effort. The effort that is lost can never be directly regained as the time that we lost is gone. Forgive everybody for everything.

We never know how much time we will have in our life so we cannot judge exactly how much we lose when we fail to be on top of our personal programming. We can optimize every facet of our lives by decisive action when re-programing seems to be needed. If we just pay attention, we can hear the guidance that comes from on high that will serve us well.

Chapter 14

Capturing Thought Patterns

Are you feeling in control of your thoughts or do they feel like they are controlling you? Either way I would invite you to start recording all troubling thoughts.

Start a Journaling process by selecting where you will assemble these notes and then just record or summarize your experience. It is a good idea to record both the date and time of each thought event and then just write freely, without editing, everything that comes to your mind.

It is most important that you capture the intensity that you felt and the emotional charge that went along with it. What was the emotion that you felt in each particular situation? Forgive everybody for everything.

Prior to the event, was there a buildup of emotions or circumstances that triggered the emotions to surge? Was there a family situation of many viewpoints that was contributory to the situation? Write it all down. Forgive everybody for everything.

Are living arrangements an irritant that makes things worse? Is work or school trouble making things worse at home? Write it all down. Forgive everybody for everything. Writing can be a continually freeing activity.

It may seem like a lot of work but real value can be had when you are able to find patterns that repeat themselves at certain intervals. Seeing the patterns can allow you to sidestep events that may trigger experiences that you might prefer to avoid. Forgive everybody for everything.

Chapter 15

Objectivity

If you feel out of control, you may benefit from a counseling session with a professional. In the past, there was stigma associated with seeking a counseling session. There are many options in today's world where you can receive wise counsel.

Perhaps one of the least threatening options for veterans now is to request an appointment with a VA chaplain. The VA has chaplains of many faiths that can sit down with you and just talk about what comes to mind. There is even a Telehealth option where technology can buffer the experience and allow an additional level of privacy.

Counselors have objectivity on their side and can sometimes see in to situations and ask precise questions that may trigger in you an awareness that you are too familiar with and cannot see. If you think of the counseling session as more of a coaching session, you may be able to psychologically sidestep any issues that you may have about counseling.

Coaching is turning in to quite a separate industry because a lot of people need to talk things out so that reality surfaces. You may be one of them and there is absolutely no shame in polishing the diamond that you are. Try to think of coaching as a way to sort out issues quickly with less personal struggle.

There is nothing like a good friend to offer objectivity when you need it. Of course, it is important to pick a friend that is not impacted directly or indirectly by the situations or people that are causing you friction.

Chapter 16

Increased Thought Intensity

As veterans, it can be that there is a level of intensity in our thoughts that can seem to be unmanageable. If that is an issue for you, I would encourage you to work on it many ways.

The most important thing is to forgive oneself. Then, seek the help that you need and be quick about it.

When the intensity of your situation is manageable again, you will have more breathing room. If you feel things are unmanageable, you need to start right away to take responsible actions to take control of your life and your feelings.

Rome was not built in a day and neither were any of the problems that you might have now. Things will not change immediately so you need to start right away and be as patient with yourself and any helpers you choose.

Forgiveness in any crisis is more important than at any other time and the forgiveness needs to include all which must include you, yourself and you.

Chapter 17

Gandhi

Gandhi said "Be the Change You Wish To See In The World" and that is still good advice.

The wise message above describes the power of taking action. Everything that is started with an idea but did not become real until action was taken to bring it into physical form

While action is important, preparation for action can help to insure that the mistakes of the past are not repeated. While you are in a reflective mood, it is important that you do your diligence to insure that the healing that you need is complete.

This is the third book in the Action Steps series and I invite you to reflect on the steps you have taken and prepare for yourself a report card. Pleas revisit the first two books and compare notes to see how you have done.

Congratulate yourself on the most important steps that you have taken to move forward with your life. Notate any issues that remain to be worked upon. Notice that the forgiveness in this book has allowed more perspective for your further healing.

Know that this reassessment is powerful insurance that you have made a solid foundation for your future growth.

Chapter 18

Your New Life Story

You may not realize it but you have accomplished a lot. Congratulations. It has taken a lot of guts for you to get this far and the cake is almost complete.

Yes, I know that you are not perfect yet and you still have some issues that need to be addressed. I also know that as long as you live there will be issues that you need to work on. Welcome back to the real world. That makes you as normal as everybody else.

It is time for you to plan the icing for your cake. What do you want to do with the rest of your life?

_____

_____

Who would you like to help you plan your life?

_____

_____

What have you dreamed about that could become a reality?

_____

_____

Chapter 19
Your New Life Plan

To claim your new life, planning can be most helpful. Take some time now to list the things that you wish to accomplish.

The goal is to balance your self-growth by intermixing the things that you want to work on (polishing points) with the sustaining needs (living essentials) you have and the dreams that tickle your heart.

Make a list of things to include in your life plan and then prioritize them and then attract them in to your reality.

Polishing Point _____

Living Essentials_____

Heart Tickle Dreams _____

Polishing Point _____

Living Essentials_____

Heart Tickle Dreams _____

Polishing Point _____

Living Essentials_____

Heart Tickle Dreams _____

Polishing Point _____

Living Essentials_____

Heart Tickle Dreams _____

Thanks for Your Service.

Thanks for Reading this far and taking care of yourself.

Thanks for any comments that you share that can help others.

May You Be Blessed AND SO IT IS!

Reverend Mike Wanner

mikewann@voicenet.com

Resource List

Distant Healing Sessions –
    Physical Healing   http://LetMeHelpYouHeal.withMike.com
    Angel Healing   http://AngelHealing.withmike.com/

Other Books by Rev. Mike at www.Amazon.com–

Trauma Healing options for VA Hospitals: Help for Veterans to Own Their Healing and their future.

Trauma Healing Action Steps For Veterans: Help To Start Healing

Trauma Healing Action Steps For Veterans: Empowerment

Trauma Healing Action Steps For Veterans: Forgiveness

Trauma Healing Action Steps For Veterans: Thought Freedom

Stress Release Energy Work: How To Cope

Angel Raphael Speaks Volume One: Take Courage! God Has Healing in Store for You

Angel Raphael Speaks Volume Two: Take Courage! God Has Healing in Store for You

Reiki Journaling From Japan

Reiki Is Alive: God's Great Gift

Four Parts To Healing

Distant Healing: We Are All Connected

Does Reiki Love Heal Cancer? : Transcribed True Stories of Spiritual Healing

Free Resources

Learn to dump fear at   http://TheGreatAmericanFearDump.withMike.com
Spiritually Prepare for Surgery   http://PrepareForSurgery.withRevMike.com
Angel Scribe messages at   http://www.SpiritualComfortCare.com
Law of Attraction Expert column at   http://www.ReverendMikeWanner.com
Stress Release at   http://www.StressReleaseCoach.com

      Angel Raphael Speaks through Rev. Mike Wanner. I have channeled multiple message sets and they all have to be polished to smooth out my errors and negotiate some words that may be too easily misunderstood. Grammar is not polished as it is too easy to miss the subtlety of the energy flow. To find out the availability of messages and latest updates go to. http://www.spiritualcomfortcare.com/angel-raphael-speaks/

Also "Tell Mike your concerns – If he and I agree there is a broader need, messages may follow. Citizens of all nations invited as long as your write in English. Do not expect him to answer as he is very busy already listening to us." E-mail Mike at mikewann@voicenet.com.

Private Channeling

Angel Raphael Speaks is a series of free messages that are channeled through Reverend Mike Wanner for the Highest good and Highest Healing of all concerned.

Many questions arise about Reverend Mike doing private channeling and he does help with that at his site http://AngelHealing.withMike.com

Reverend Mike is available world-wide as a psychic channel, emotional release facilitator, spiritual energy practitioner & teacher, and public speaker.

He looks forward to meeting you soon!

Email - mikewann@voicenet.com 215-342-1270 http://AngelHealing.withMike.com

PRIVATE SPIRITUAL READINGS/channelings or Spiritual Healing Sessions: Telephone or in person

Rev. Mike is available for private, one-on-one intuitive sessions with you, his Guide Family, and your Guides. He helps by offering clarity on emotional situations about your life, your purpose, your spirituality, and the release of stuffed emotions and cellular memory.

Connect to the love of your Guides today! Contact Rev. Mike for an appointment.

Go to the page – http://AngelHealing.withMike.com

Sessions available:

1. Spiritual Readings
2. Angel Channeling
3. Distant Reiki Healing
4. Distant Clearing of Stuffed Emotions
5. Distant Clearing of Cellular Memory
6. Distant Clearing of Energy Blockages
7. Distant Clearing of the Chakras
8. Mastermind dowsing responses to yes/no direction finding questions.
9. Customized needs

Rev. Mike is a facilitator of healing. He brings you and the Divine together so that you can align with the Divine and have a great time and a great life. All healing is between you and God, as it should be.

Rev. Michael Wanner

Rev. Michael Wanner started his metaphysical and ministerial studies with Reiki in 1993 and has studied seven styles of Reiki in the U.S., Japan, Canada, Denmark and Australia. He is certified to teach. He became certified to teach Integrated Energy Therapy in 1999 and co-taught the first IET class of the new Millennium. Mike began dowsing in 2001.

Ordained as a Metaphysical Minister of the International Metaphysical Ministry and an Interfaith Minister of the Circle of Miracles Ministry, Rev. Mike practices and teaches spiritual energy therapies in the Philadelphia Area.

Rev. Mike holds ministerial degrees from the University of Metaphysics and the University of Sedona. He is a Pastoral Care Associate of Aria – Frankford Hospital. He taught at the National Academy of Massage Therapy and Health Sciences.

Rev. Mike was a faculty member of the Medical Mission Sister's Center for Human Integration's School of Integrated Body/Mind Therapies in Fox Chase, Philadelphia, PA for twelve years.

Rev. Mike is licensed by the teaching of Intuitional Metaphysics to practice Spiritual Healing and Scientific Prayer. Mike is also a Prayer therapist.

Rev. Mike was elected in 2007 to the status of "Fellow of the American Institute of Stress."

In 2008, Rev. Mike became a practitioner of Coincidental Recognition as he incorporated the CoRe system in to his spiritual healing practice.

In 2009, Rev. Mike trademarked a new healing process called Quantum Quatro! Subtle Energy System Support®.

In 2011, Rev. Mike joined the outreach program known as the Health Advantage Group.

In 2012. Rev. Mike became a Certified Professional Coach by The Master Coaching Academy and Joined The Personal Empowerment Group .

Prior to his metaphysical, ministerial and coaching studies, Rev. Mike worked for Sears Roebuck and Co. while in High School and after graduation until he joined the U. S. Air Force in 1965. He returned to Sears from Vietnam in 1969 and stayed until 1978. His final Sears assignment was as an efficiency expert in Methods - Operational Research and Development.

He volunteered with Burholme Emergency Medical Services from 1969 and is still a Life Member and Board of Directors Member. He started a private ambulance company in 1975 and worked professionally in the field until 2001 when he devoted his full attention to real estate investing, healing and coaching.